Soumaya Smaali
Amine Trabelsi
Seif Hannechi

Spirulina

AF536095

Soumaya Smaali
Amine Trabelsi
Seif Hannechi

Spirulina

Production, Quality Control and Jobs

ScienciaScripts

Imprint

Any brand names and product names mentioned in this book are subject to trademark, brand or patent protection and are trademarks or registered trademarks of their respective holders. The use of brand names, product names, common names, trade names, product descriptions etc. even without a particular marking in this work is in no way to be construed to mean that such names may be regarded as unrestricted in respect of trademark and brand protection legislation and could thus be used by anyone.

Cover image: www.ingimage.com

This book is a translation from the original published under ISBN 978-620-6-72792-7.

Publisher:
Sciencia Scripts
is a trademark of
Dodo Books Indian Ocean Ltd. and OmniScriptum S.R.L publishing group

120 High Road, East Finchley, London, N2 9ED, United Kingdom
Str. Armeneasca 28/1, office 1, Chisinau MD-2012, Republic of Moldova, Europe
Managing Directors: Ieva Konstantinova, Victoria Ursu
info@omniscriptum.com

Printed at: see last page
ISBN: 978-620-8-54519-2

Copyright © Soumaya Smaali, Amine Trabelsi, Seif Hannechi
Copyright © 2025 Dodo Books Indian Ocean Ltd. and OmniScriptum S.R.L publishing group

CONTENTS

LIST OF ABBREVIATIONS

ALAT: Alanine aminotransferase

ANSES: Agence nationale de sécurité de l'alimentation, de l'environnement et du travail (French Agency for Food, Environmental and Occupational Safety)

ANSM : Agence nationale de sécurité du médicament et des produits de santé

ASAT: Aspartate aminotransferase

EABA*: European Algae Biomass Association*

EFSA*: European Food Safety Authority*

ELISA: *Enzyme-linked immunosorbent* assay

EMA: *European medicines agency*

EPS: Exopolysaccharide

FAO: Food and Agriculture Organization of the United Nations

FDA: *Food and Drug* Administration

GRAS: "*Generally Recognized As Safe*

PAH: Polycyclic aromatic hydrocarbon

LDH: Lactate

WHO: World Health Organization

SEMC: Southern and Eastern Mediterranean Countries

USP: *Dietary Supplements Compendium*

WHO: *World Heath Organization*

INTRODUCTION

Microalgae are among the most promising renewable raw materials for healthy, functional food products.

Microalgae contain a number of bioactive compounds that can meet people's nutrient and energy needs, and boost immunity to prevent chronic disease.

Various processes have demonstrated the potential of these microorganisms in the cosmetics and food industries, and in the production of pigments and additives. Microalgae need no arable land and can use waste products as nutrients for growth. Several species thrive in extreme environments, so their production processes are increasingly being described .**[1]**

Among them spirulina, a blue-green algae. Spirulina is a photosynthetic filamentous cyanobacteria known for biomass production due to its high cell growth rate, ease of harvesting and potential market as a human or veterinary food supplement.

Spirulina has a high protein content, a unique composition of fatty acids, pigments (phycocyanin and β-carotene) and a high carbohydrate content. In addition, this microalgae contains up to 70% protein and has interesting nutritional properties thanks to its content of essential amino acids, vitamins and minerals.

Today, this cyanobacteria appears to be an interesting solution for large-scale industries to produce a top-quality food supplement. As result, spirulina cultivation on an industrial scale is booming. In addition to its proven nutritional qualities, spirulina is now attracting the interest of the international scientific community for its pharmaceutical and nutraceutical potential .**[2]**

It has therapeutic properties thanks to its functional compounds, such as phenolics, phycocyanins and polysaccharides, with antioxidant, anti-inflammatory and immunostimulant effects .**[3]**

This led us to take an interest in the subject and devote this book to it, whose objectives are first to define spirulina and show its richness in nutrients. Next, we'll explain the various stages of cultivation and production parameters at both artisanal and industrial levels. Next, we'll present the trials and tests carried out on spirulina in the various monographs, with the aim of controlling the quality of this microalga so as to obtain a high-quality product that meets international standards. Finally, we'll look at the uses and side effects associated with spirulina consumption.

1. PRESENTATION OF SPIRULINA

1.1.History

Spirulina is the oldest living plant on Earth**[4]** . It used to be classified as blue-green algae. Strictly speaking, it is not an alga, although it continues to be referred to as such**[5]** . Blue-green algae are cyanobacteria: an evolutionary bridge between bacteria and green plants**[4]**

Spirulina was first discovered by Spanish scientist Hernando Cortez in 1519. He observed spirulina being eaten at Aztec tables during his visit to Lake Texcoco in the Valley of Mexico **[1]**. Microalgae gathered on the shores of lakes are harvested, then sun-dried and molded into small bricks, then dried in thin layers before consumption .**[6]**

Pierre Dangeard, a French botanist and mycologist, discovered that the Kanembou populations living around Lake Chad in Africa harvested *Arthrospira platensis* for use as a food called "*Dihé*". In a study describing how the Kanembou used this seaweed, Delpeuch *et al.* (1976) found that the main use was as a sauce accompanying meals, and that direct consumption of dried "*Dihé*" cookies only occurred for superstitious reasons among pregnant women, since its dark color would protect the unborn baby from the evil of sorcerers, according to a popular local belief. *Arthrospira* from Lake Chad is still harvested and used today, as shown in **figure 1[7]**

We're talking here about a major impact on the population's standard of living, not to mention the as yet unassessed impact on health**[5]**

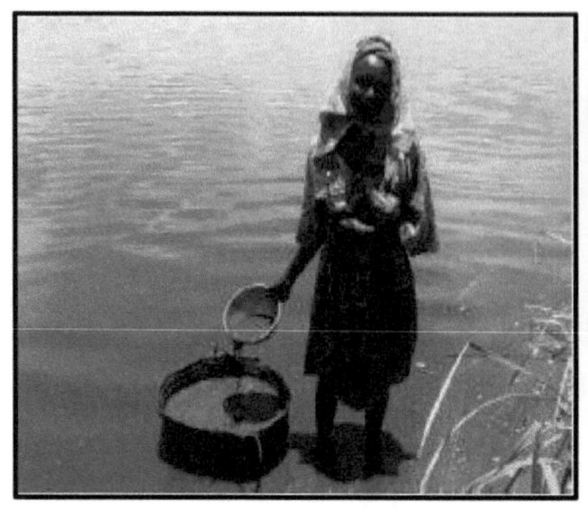 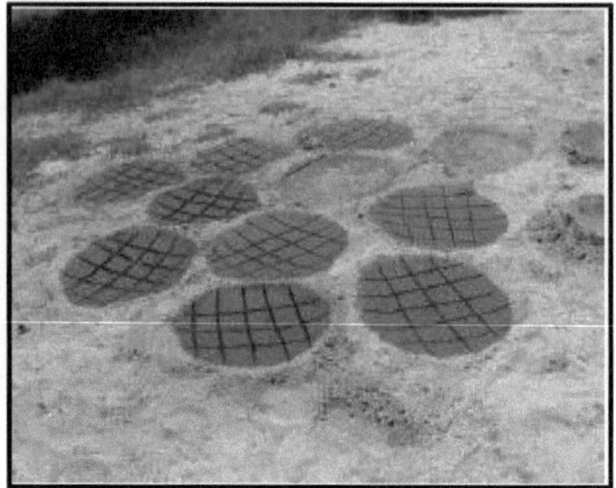

Figure 1: Traditional spirulina harvesting and drying in Lake Chad .[7]

1.2.Classification and geographical distribution

Spirulina is a Gram-negative cyanobacterium. Generally speaking, cyanobacteria are either unicellular or multicellular.

Taxonomically, spirulina is classified in the order Oscillatoriales, family Microcoleaceae , genus *Arthrospira.*

Spirulina thrives best in warm, alkaline waters rich in nitrogen and phosphorus nutrients. It is more commonly found in brackish waters, but also in saline lakes in tropical and semi-tropical zones. Spirulina is thermophilic and needs a lot of light, which limits its range to a well-defined region of the globe, from 35° south latitude to 35° north latitude.

Spirulina is characterized by a strong ability to maintain its wild phenotype despite considerable environmental variations; this allows it to survive in its natural state in alkaline lakes on 3 continents: Africa (Tunisia, Chad), South Asia (Sri Lanka) and Latin America (Peru)... etc. It is therefore said to be ubiquitous, although much less abundant in the northern regions of the world. It is therefore said to be ubiquitous, although much less abundant in the northern regions of the globe .**[8]**

1.3.Morphology and general characteristics

Spirulina has an average size around 250µm. Its structure is characterized by filaments no more than 12 microns in diameter.

These are simple (unbranched) and generally wound into 6 or 7 coils. It's these spirals, giving the cyanobacteria a spring-like appearance, have earned spirulina its name.

However, spirulina are not homomorphic. As shown in **Figure 2**, they include the spiral forms already described, as well as wavy and sometimes straight forms. This heteromorphism is directly linked to the ecological conditions encountered in their habitat .**[8]**

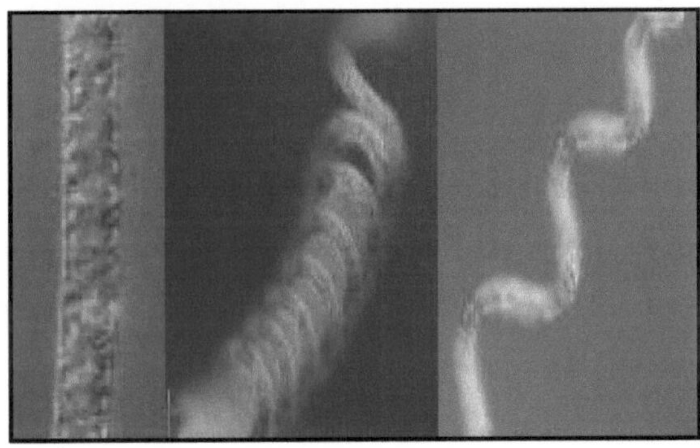

Figure 2: The different forms of spirulina .[9]

1.4.Reproduction

Spirulina has a simple life cycle. It is illustrated schematically **in Figure 3**.

When spirulina filaments reach maturity, special cyanobacterial cells called necridia appear. These differ from "normal" cells in their biconcave appearance, and form separation discs. From these, the trichome splits to form hormogonia, made up of 2 to 4 cells. Through scissiparity (binary division), the hormogonia grow in length and take on the typical helical shape. In vitro, spirulina has a maximum generation time of around 7 hours .**[10]**

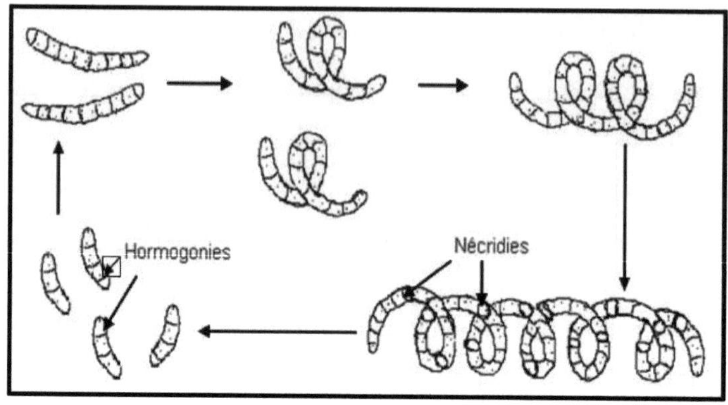

Figure 3: Spirulina life cycle .[8]

1.5.Composition

1.5.1.

Spirulina is known for its high protein content: 10% of its wet mass, equivalent to almost 65% of its dry mass. This significantly exceeds the protein content of foods known to be rich in protein: 35% for milk powder, 25% for blue fish and only 14% for cereals .**[11]**

However, the protein content of spirulina varies from 10 to 15% depending on harvesting time and photoperiod. The highest levels are found at the beginning of the light period. These values may also vary according to the drying processes used .**[12]**

Spirulina has a polysaccharide envelope rather than a cellulose wall. This low cellulose content makes it highly digestible even without cooking**[13]**

Spirulina's proteins are virtually complete. Several essential amino acids are present, accounting for 47% of the total weight **[5]** . **Table I** shows the various amino acids and their content per 100g of spirulina.

Table I: Amino acid content per 100g of spirulina .[3]

Amino acids	Amino acid content per 100g of spirulina
Leucine	5.9-8.4 g
Aspartate	5.2-6.0 g
Lysine	2.6-4.6 g
Phenylalanine	2.6-4.1 g
Tyrosine	2.6-3.4 g
Methionine	1.3-2.7 g

1.5.2. Lipids

Seven percent of spirulina's dry weight corresponds to lipids. There are two lipid fractions: a saponifiable fraction (83%) and an unsaponifiable fraction (17%). A good balance between saturated and polyunsaturated fatty acids characterizes the total lipid composition.

Fatty acids (saponifiable fraction) make up 4.9 to 5.7% of spirulina dry matter, and are mainly represented by phosphatidyl glycerol (25.9%), mono- and di-galactosyl diglyceride (23%), and sulfoquinovosyl diglyceride (5%) .**[8]**

Li, Tian-Tian et al. described the composition of the main fatty acids in 3 spirulina species (*S. pacifica, S. maxima, S. platensis*) as being marked by a high concentration of essential fatty acids (unsaturated fatty acids), including omega-3 and omega-6 .**[14]**

Gamma-linolenic acid constitutes up to 40% of fatty acids in *S. platensis* (or 4% of dry weight) and 10 to 20% (or 1-2% of dry weight) in *S. maxima.* The presence of gamma-linolenic acid is noteworthy given the rarity of this compound in common foods, and its role as a precursor of chemical mediators of inflammatory and immune reactions .**[15]**

Sterols, saturated hydrocarbons (kerosenes), terpenes and pigments form the unsaponifiable fraction, which accounts for 1.2% of spirulina dry matter .**[8]**

1.5.3. Carbohydrates

Thirteen to 25% of spirulina dry matter consists of carbohydrates. The cyanobacterial wall is made up of glucosamine and muramic acid combined with peptides, as in Gram-negative bacteria.

Assimilable carbohydrates are essentially polymers, mainly glucosan and rhamnosan. Water-extractable mucilage makes up around 11% of spirulina's dry weight.

Cyclitols account for 3% of cyanobacterial dry matter and are present in phosphorylated form. Their main compounds are meso-inositol phosphate (source of organic phosphorus) and inositol (350-850mg dry matter) .**[10]**

1.5.4. Vitamins

Spirulina contains a variety of water- and fat-soluble vitamins in very interesting quantities, as shown in **Table II**.

Table II: Vitamin content in µg/g spirulina dry matter .[8]

Vitamin	Content	Vitamin	Content
Water-soluble vitamins		Fat-soluble vitamins	
B1 (thiamine)	34-50	Provitamin A (β-carotene)	700-1700
B2 (riboflavin)	30-46	Cryptoxanthin	100
B3 (niacin)	130	Vitamin E (α-tocopherol)	120
B5 (pantothenate)	4,6-25		
B6 (pyridoxine)	5-8		
B8 (biotin)	0,05		
B9 (folate)	0,5		
B12 (cobalamin)	0.10-0.34		
C (ascorbic acid)	Traces		

1.5.5. Minerals and trace elements

Spirulina is a source of various minerals, as shown in **Table III**.

Table III: Mineral composition of cultivated spirulina in µg/g dry matter .[10]

Minerals	Content
Calcium	1300-14000
Phosphorus	6700-9000
Magnesium	2000-2900
Iron	580-1800
Zinc	21-40
Copper	8-10
Chrome	2,8
Manganese	25-37
Sodium	4500
Potassium	6400-15400

1.5.6. Functional compounds

One of the reasons why spirulina is such an exceptional food source is its content of functional compounds, grouped in **Table IV**.

Table IV: Content of functional compounds per 100g of spirulina .[3]

Functional compounds	Content in g/100g of spirulina
Phenolic compounds	0.20 - 1.73
Flavonoids	0.1 - 0.9
Phycocyanins C	13.5 - 14.8
Allophycocyanin	2.3
Phycobiliproteins	1.1
Polysaccharides	0.2 - 12.5
β-carotenes	0.008

1.5.6.1. Polyphenolic compounds

Polyphenolic compounds include benzophenone, dihydro-methyl-phenylacridine, carbanilic acid, dinitrobenzoate, propanediamine, isoquinoline, piperidine, oxazolidine and pyrrolidine .**[16]**

The antimicrobial effect of phenolic compounds can be exploited to preserve foods, and some of these compounds could be used in several fields (food industry, pharmaceuticals, cosmetics). Some studies report that phenolic compounds have powerful antioxidant properties due to their ability to scavenge free radicals via hydroxyl groups .**[17]**

1.5.6.2. Pigments

The main pigment classes in microalgae are carotenoids and phycobiliproteins**[1]** . Phycobiliproteins are a group of highly water-soluble proteins covalently linked to chromophores, which are open-chain tetrapyrroles, also known as phycobilins. These molecules possess chromophores responsible for coloration (**Figure 4**).

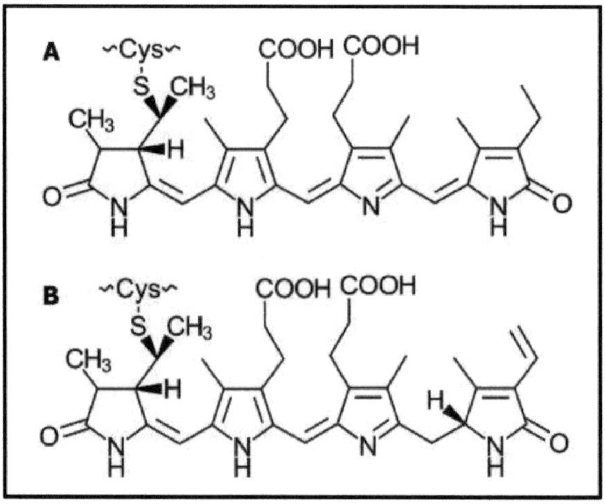

Figure 4: Chemical structures of phycocyanin (A) and phycoerythrin (B)[18] .

These protein complexes have been named for their optical properties: phycoerythrins (λ_{max}= 565 nm), phycocyanins (λ_{max}= 618 nm) and allophycocyanin (λ_{max}= 655 nm). In addition to chlorophyll, these pigments capture the light energy required for photosynthesis .**[19]**

Phycocyanin is an immune stimulant. It acts at bone marrow level by stimulating and regulating the evolution and differentiation of stem cells of the erythroblastic and granular lineages .**[20]**

Recent studies also suggest that spirulina has anti-inflammatory activity, which may be due to the selective inhibition of cyclooxygenase type 2 and the efficient scavenging of free radicals, which opposes lipid peroxidation**[21]** and may explain the hepatoprotective, anti-inflammatory and anti-arthritic properties .**[22]**

1.5.6.3. Membrane polysaccharides

Spirulina's shell is composed of polysaccharides bearing sulfated residues and consisting of mannose, galactose, glucose, rhamnose, fructose, xylose, ribose, galacturonic and glucuronic acids, as well as calcium and sodium ions**[23]** . These natural polymers present themselves as a promising biomaterial, as they are safe, non-toxic and biodegradable. Thus, the synthesis of micro- and nanoparticles from polysaccharides for industrial purposes in the fields of pharmaceutical, cosmetic and food engineering has been studied .**[24]**

Membrane polysaccharides are also capable of stimulating the immune system at humoral level through the production of cytokines and antibodies, and at cellular level through the mobilization of T lymphocytes, macrophages and NK cells

Membrane polysaccharides are also involved in the stimulation of endonucleases. Endonucleases are involved in the repair of genome damage, such as that caused by radiotoxic or chemotoxic substances, and thus prevent oncogenesis .**[20]**

2. SPIRULINA PRODUCTION

Spirulina is produced in a number of ways: artisanal, semi-industrial and industrial. These production scales differ in terms of the surface area allocated to cultivation ponds and their unit surface areas, the technology used, and the means and materials employed. However, similar compulsory stages are followed whatever the manufacturing process.

Spirulina is grown on an industrial scale in countries such as the USA, Thailand and India. Family or artisanal farming is found in African countries (Burkina Faso, Senegal, Togo, etc.).

The culture medium must be enriched with nutrients, with adjusted pH and salinity .**[8]**

2.1.Cropping systems

2.1.1. Open cropping systems

The cultivation of algae in open culture systems has been extensively studied in recent years. These systems can be classified into natural (lakes, lagoons, etc.) and artificial cultivation environments .**[25]**

Raceway" type ponds have been the most widely used since they first appeared in the 50s. They are based on the circulation of algae at shallow widths and depths (between 15 and 50 cm) but over long distances, as shown in **figure 5**. Low-energy paddlewheels ensure circulation and mixing. These basins have a productivity of around 20 g/m^2/d, for a cell concentration of less than 0.6 g/l .**[26]**

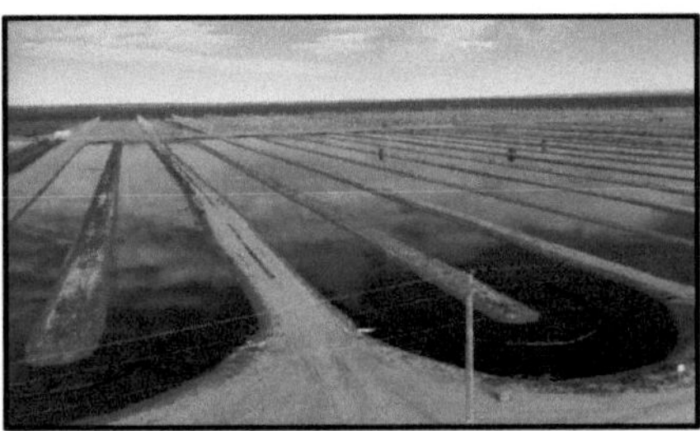

Figure 5: Open *raceway* spirulina cultivation system[27]

There are several ways to build a suitable pond, depending on the ambient conditions.

Sharp corners should be avoided in the design of the pond, in favor of rounded corners. The edges of the pond, at least 20 to 40 cm above the bottom, should extend above ground level, to avoid contamination by animal waste and dust.

Ponds can be made of plastic sheeting, concrete, cinder blocks, bricks, galvanized steel or, more rarely, clay. For small-scale production, the total surface area of ponds should not exceed 300 m^2 .**[28]**

It is often necessary to install a roof or, preferably, a greenhouse to protect the pond from falling leaves and waste, and from excessive sun, rain or cold. The design of open-roof greenhouses offers complete protection against undesirable weather conditions**[4]**

2.1.2. Closed cultivation systems

Photobioreactors are made of transparent materials.

In order to achieve maximum productivity, we focus on controlling cultivation parameters (temperature, carbon dioxide, oxygen and pH), as well as illuminated surface area and mixing efficiency.

Photobioreactors come in many forms: flat photobioreactors, cylindrical photobioreactors and sheath-type photobioreactors .**[29]**

2.1.2.1. Flat photobioreactors

Flat photobioreactors are no more than 10 cm thick. This minimizes the light path. Generally speaking, the thinner the culture, the higher the productivity. **Figure 6** shows these photobioreactors. They can be arranged horizontally or vertically, with a degree of inclination to maximize incident light intensity. Polymer honeycomb plates or glass panels can be used .**[29]**

These photobioreactors require less feeding than tubular photobioreactors to achieve sufficient mass and heat transfer capacity. However, aeration stress has sometimes been reported in these photobioreactors, whereas it has never been reported in tubular photobioreactors. In both cases, knowledge of the reactor's heat transfer capacity enables the correct design of heat storage systems, thus considerably improving the system's energy efficiency .**[30]**

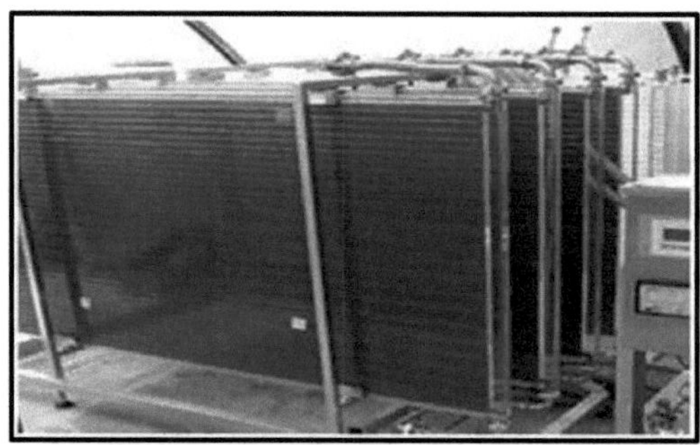

Figure 6: Planar photobioreactors .[4]

2.1.2.2. Cylindrical photobioreactors

- **Column type**

Small-scale microalgae production is generally associated with this type of reactor (**figure 7**). They come in a variety of forms, from simple bubble columns to annular photobioreactors, not forgetting air circulation photobioreactors or "*Airlifts*".

Vertical column photobioreactors are compact, inexpensive and easy to operate and sterilize, with low energy consumption. But they also have drawbacks: their construction requires sophisticated materials and they have a small illumination surface .**[25]**

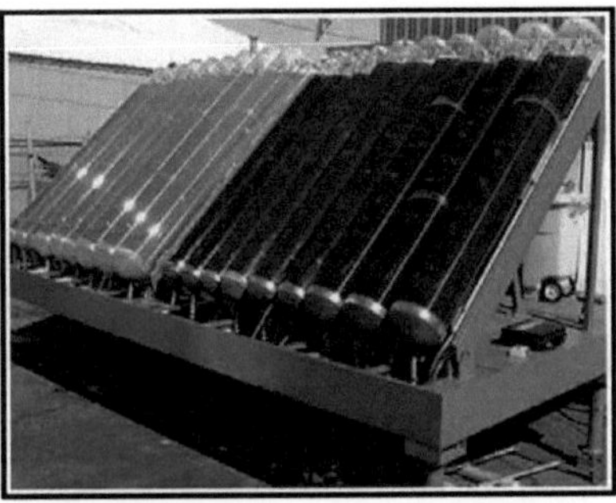

Figure 7: Column-type photobioreactors .[4]

- **Tubular type**

These tubes are often made of glass or plastic, with diameters ranging from just 2 to 6 cm, to allow light to reach the center of the crop. They can be very long, and are arranged horizontally or vertically in the form of coils, and wound helically. **Figure 8** shows two different forms of this type of photobioreactor. For structural reasons, they are limited to a height of 4 meters. Lighting is provided by fluorescent tubes or, failing that, by simple exposure to the sun**[29]**
The disadvantages of this type of photobioreactor are the accumulation of oxygen, the occupation of a large surface area and a very high construction cost .**[31]**

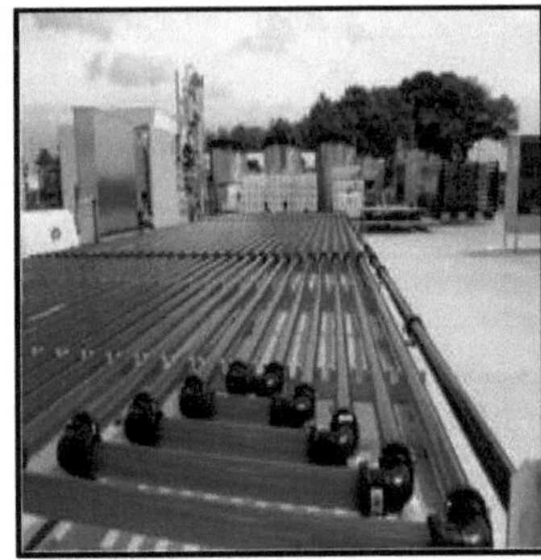

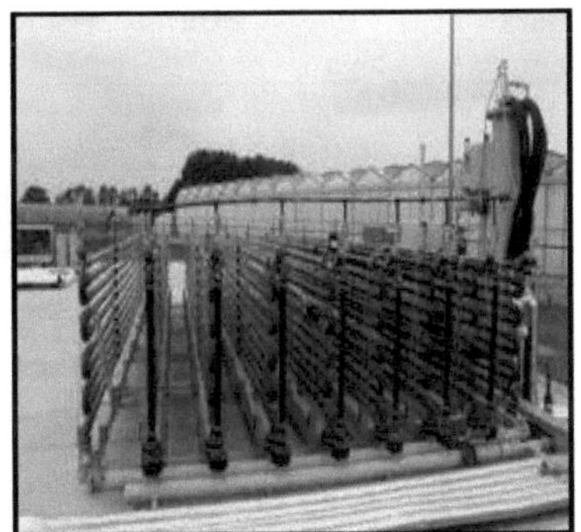

Figure 8Horizontal and vertical tubular photobioreactors .[32]

2.1.2.3. Duct-type photobioreactor

This model uses polyethylene sheaths, suspended by their ends from a metal support, as shown in **figure 9** below, and generally lit by neon lamps. This system is relatively popular, thanks to its simplicity and ease of use. The bag can be easily replaced when excessive clogging or contamination occurs .**[30]**

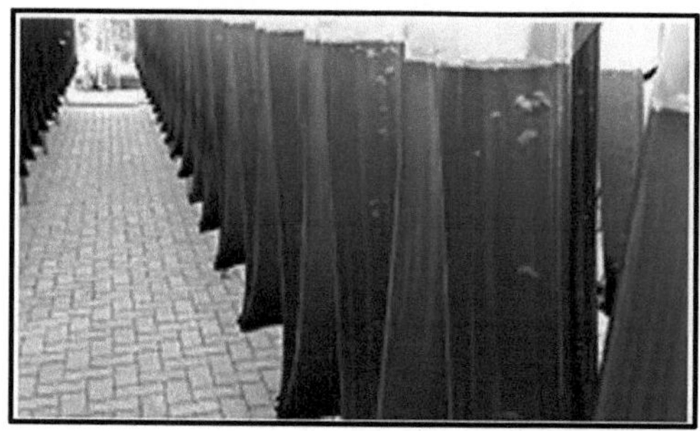

Figure 9: Duct-type photobioreactors .[4]

2.1.3. Comparison

Following the description of the two types of cropping systems, a comparison of their advantages and disadvantages seems necessary (**Table V**).

Table V: Comparison between an open cultivation system (ponds) and photobioreactors .[33]

Factors	Basins	Photobioreactors
Space required	high	low
Water loss	Very high, can also cause salt precipitation	Low
Loss of CO(2	High, depending on pool depth	Low
Oxygen concentration	Usually low	Accumulation in a closed system requires gas exchange devices (O_2 must be eliminated to avoid inhibition of photosynthesis and photo-oxidation).
Temperature	Highly variable, some control possible depending on pool depth	Cooling often required (by immersing tubes in cooling baths)

Risk of contamination	High (limiting the number of species that can be grown)	Medium to low
Biomass quality	Variable	Reproducible
Biomass concentration	Low 0.1-0.5 g/l	High, 0.5-8.0 g/l
Production flexibility	Few possible species, difficult to change	High, change possible
Process control and reproducibility	Limited	Possible
dependency	High (precipitation, light intensity, temperature)	Medium (light intensity, cooling required)
Start	6 to 8 weeks	2 to 4 weeks
Operating costs	Low (impeller, addition of CO_2)	Higher costs ($CO_{(2)}$) addition, oxygen removal, cooling, cleaning, maintenance)
Harvesting costs	High, species-dependent	Lower due to high biomass concentration and better control of species and conditions

2.2.Culture media

2.2.1. Zarrouk" midfield

This is a standard medium which can even be used as a reference. It uses distilled water and contains several reagents, as shown in **Tables VI** and **VII**. This medium is often cited, even though it's not very economical.

Table VI: Composition of the "Zarrouk" medium in g/l .[28]

Composition	Concentration	Composition	Concentration
$NaHCO_3$	16,8	$CaCl_2$	0,04
K_2HPO_4	0,5	$FeSO_4$, 7 H_2O	0,01
$NaNO_3$	2,5	EDTA	0,08
K_2SO_4	1	solution A5, solution B6	2 (50/50)
NaCl	1	$MgSO_4$, 7 H_2O	0,2

Table VII: Composition of medium A5 and B6 in g/l .[28]

Solution A5		Solution B6	
Composition	**Concentration**	**Composition**	**Concentration**
H_3BO_3	2,86	NH_4VO_3	0,02296
$MnCl_2$, 4 H_2O	1,81	$K_2Cr_2(SO_4)_4$, 24 H_2O	0,096
$ZnSO_4$, 7 H_2O	0,222	$NiSO_4$, 7 H_2O	0,04785
$CuSO_4$, 5 H_2O	0,079	Na_2WO_4, 2 H_2O	0,01794
MoO_3	0,015	$Ti_2(SO_4)_3$	0,04
		$Co(NO_3)2$,6 H_2O	0,04398

2.2.2. Example of a more economical environment

In mass spirulina cultivation, nutritional status is one of the main factors influencing growth and productivity. Simple means are needed to reduce the cost of large-scale spirulina production. This intention has been implemented by replacing all the nutrients in the "Zarrouk" medium with cheaper commercial fertilizers and chemicals.

The low-cost medium contains :

- Single super-phosphate: 1.25 g/l
- Commercial sodium bicarbonate: 16.8 g/l
- Muriate of potash: 0.898 g/l
- Raw sea salt: 1 g/l
- ammonium nitrate or urea (the nitrogen concentration can vary from 10 to 40% of the nitrogen concentration of the "Zarrouk" medium) .**[34]**

2.2.3. Example of a more ecological environment

The production of fungal biomass from *Aspergillus niger* was carried out using media composed of wheat bran and/or potato peel. The fungal biomass was used as a bio-flocculant in cultures produced in 5 L closed reactors and in a 180 L open "*Raceway*" tank operating in batch and semi-batch mode respectively. The fungal biomass was able to generate *Spirulina platensis* cultures with efficiencies of between 90% and 100% after 2 h of sedimentation. Yields> 80% were obtained in most tests without pH adjustment during bioflocculation, demonstrating that the method developed is a promising alternative to traditional spirulina harvesting techniques [ ] .**19**

2.3.Craft production

In Chad, traditional "*Dihé*" spirulina production involves two essential stages: harvesting and drying.

Initially, the product is collected in basins and cups. Then, to eliminate the water, the product obtained is introduced into sand trays. After two or three days, the product becomes dry, with a thickness of no more than 8 cm.

However, this result is far from perfect. There are several types of contaminants: sand (> 30%), plant, insect and animal debris.

This increases the risk of transmission of pathogens and food poisoning

The presence of sand also makes it necessary to boil the "*Dihé*" before consumption. It's worth mentioning that this traditional dish is generally served in sauces, which require a lot of time and steps to prepare (around 2 to 3 cookings), resulting in a marked reduction in nutrients, especially heat-sensitive proteins and vitamins.

A simple, accessible process has now been introduced to remedy these problems, comprising the following stages: : Harvesting, sieving, pre-concentration, extrusion, drying, grinding and packaging.

The products obtained are in the form of spaghetti, cake, powder or capsule, with a blue-green color close to that of fresh "*Dihé*". They are of superior quality and free from impurities. These products can be eaten fresh or dried, without cooking, which preserves their nutrients. .**[7]**

2.3.1. Seeding

If cultivation is carried out in tanks, the first step would be to select the strain using a microscope or magnifying glass. In order to guarantee a safe stock, it is advisable to carry out this examination regularly. .**[28]**

Different strains exist, although they all share common characteristics that differentiate them from other cyanobacteria. **Table VIII** shows the differences between wavy and spiral strains

Although "spiralized" ones look better under the microscope, in practice, "wavy" ones are preferred.

Table VIII: Differences between wavy and spiral strains[36]

Spirals	The wavy ones
▪ Their greater buoyancy than corrugated and straight lines allows them to be separated. ▪ Easier biomass drying. ▪ Not pump-resistant ▪ At low pH and in the absence of ammonium, they form floating lumps.	▪ Under normal conditions, they do not tend to become straight. ▪ Resistant to pumping (by centrifugal pump) and osmotic shock (can be washed with fresh water). ▪ Not suspected of being "fake" spirulina.

To start a culture, we recommend starting the highest possible spirulina concentrations and ensuring a level of 5 to 10 cm of liquid

The spirulina is placed in the first tank for two weeks, before being transferred to another medium-sized tank and finally to a larger tank, where it is supplied with sodium bicarbonate and potassium. Cultivation generally takes 6 months to reach maturity, as indicated by the green color of the water**[37]**

2.3.2. Harvest

Daily harvesting of one-sixth to one-third of the culture is possible under optimal conditions. The culture is filtered through two superimposed meshes of decreasing mesh size (from 300 μm to 30 μm).

The first device (fine mesh) retains larvae, insects, leaves and lumps, while the second retains spirulina.

Fresh, moist spirulina is pressed and can be eaten as is or stored after drying.**[7]**

Managing crop concentration is crucial. A high concentration without harvesting can be lethal for the biomass. However, a concentration below 0.4 g/l makes the crop less stable, although productivity is higher at lower concentrations. .**[28]**

2.3.3. Drying and packaging

For easy and efficient drying, the biomass is transformed into spaghetti using an extruder. **Figure 10** shows the resulting shape. It is placed in gas, solar or electric dryers**[7]** . The dried material thus obtained is then reduced to powder or flakes and stored in an airtight container, protected from light and humidity. .**[28]**

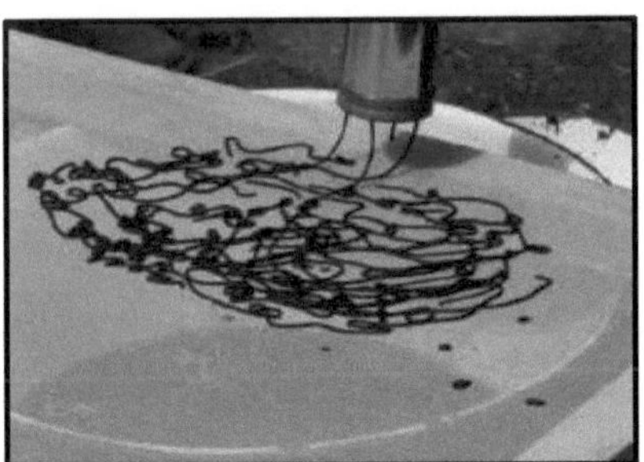

Figure 10: Biomass is extruded into spaghetti .[7]

2.4.Industrial production

Commercial spirulina production involves four stages: cultivation, harvesting, drying and packaging. All these stages can affect final yield and product quality. Careful and regular monitoring of these processes is therefore essential to the successful production of high-quality spirulina that meets the international safety and quality requirements of the food and dietary supplement industry**[38]**

2.4.1. Harvest

The best time to harvest is early in the morning for the following reasons:

- Protein levels are highest in the morning.
- The cool temperature makes work easier.
- More hours of sunlight will be available to dry the product.

The various harvesting techniques used are: filtration, flotation, centrifugation, precipitation and ultrasonic vibration .**[4]**

2.4.1.1. Centrifugation

The aim is to separate the spirulina from the culture medium. Centrifugation or chemical precipitation are economically feasible, but centrifugation is more sensitive. This method is reasonably efficient, but sensitive strains can be damaged by granulation against the rotor wall .**[4]**

2.4.1.2. Filtration

Filtration produces a biomass containing around 10% dry matter and 50% residual culture medium. A filter or mesh of at least 50 microns is used to collect the spirulina efficiently

There are two types of sieves: inclined sieves and vibrating sieves.

The inclined screens measure 380 to 500 mesh with a filtration area of 2 to 4 m^2 per unit and are capable of harvesting around 10 to 18 m^3 of spirulina culture per hour. Biomass harvesting efficiency is very high, close to 95%. A fixed, inclined sieve is considered a better solution for harvesting spirulina. Vibrating sieves filter the same volume per unit time as inclined sieves. The combination of an inclined filter and a vibrating sieve is possible**[4]**

2.4.2. Drying and packaging

The paste obtained from the filtered spirulina is washed three times with water to remove the salt before entering a drying vessel which converts it to powder. The dried spirulina flakes are ground using a high-impact ultra-fine grinder. Grinding continues for around 6-10 h, until the average powder size reaches 200-800 nm. Powder and tablets are the most common forms of spirulina available on the market. The powder is generally blue-green in color, as shown in **figure 11 .[4]**

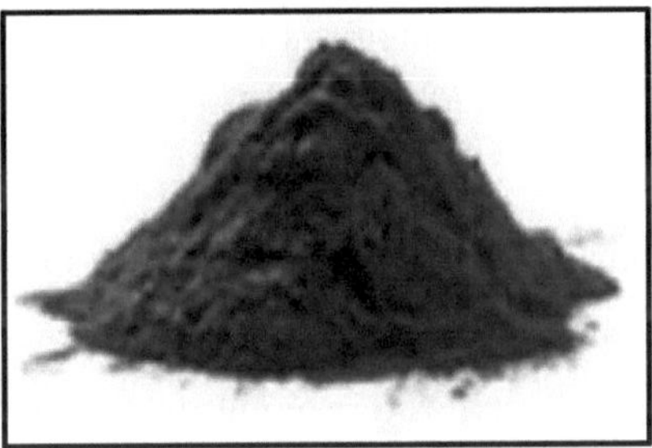

Figure 11: Spirulina powder .[39]

It is pressed into a kind of tablet or granule for better acceptability and performance. **Figure 12** shows the appearance of these tablets

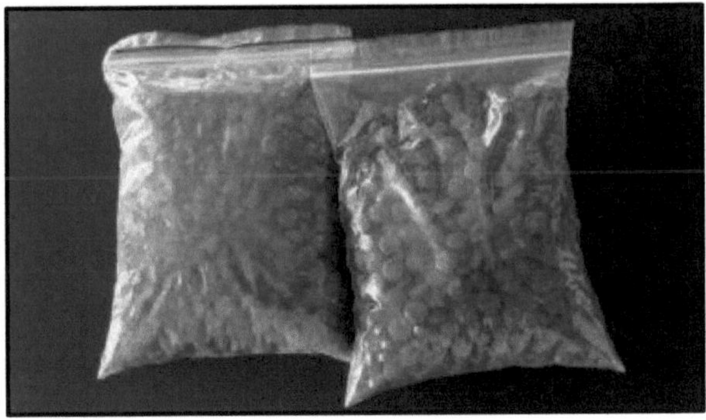

Figure 12: Spirulina tablets .[40]

The advantages of spirulina granules are as follows.

- Excellent water stability
- Easy consumption
- Longer shelf life.

No preservatives, additives or stabilizers are used .**[4]**

Appropriate packaging is also important for high-quality spirulina production. The dried powder is weighed and vacuum-sealed in airtight bags to minimize exposure to air and prevent possible oxidation of the light-sensitive nutrients. The bags are then packed in cardboard boxes sealed with tape and labeled to reflect package weight and batch numbers for tracking purposes. All necessary preventive measures are taken to ensure that production procedures do not contribute to contamination of the processed product by harmful chemicals, undesirable micro-organisms or any other undesirable material. Following these packaging parameters, the product can remain fresh for up to four years with little change in biochemical composition or nutritional properties .**[38]**

2.5.Influential factors and production optimization

Microalgae growth and production are part of a complex photosynthetic process with multiple influencing factors such as water, nutrient conditions, light, pH, and temperature. These various factors can trigger critical situations that could damage cultivation and biomass harvesting. Dangerous situations for the crop must be controlled, anticipated and avoided**[26]**

2.5.1. Light

The key factor in spirulina's photosynthetic growth is light.

At low light intensities, the rate of photosynthesis is proportional to light intensity. However, at high light intensities, photosynthesis increases until it reaches a maximum level. This photo-limitation results in low biomass productivity, particularly in open ponds. **Figure 13** clearly shows this plateau in the second segment of the curve. Photo-limitation can be reduced by decreasing the depth of cultivation**[41]**

Another phenomenon also observed at high light intensities: photo-inhibition, where excess light reduces the rate of photosynthesis. .**[29]**

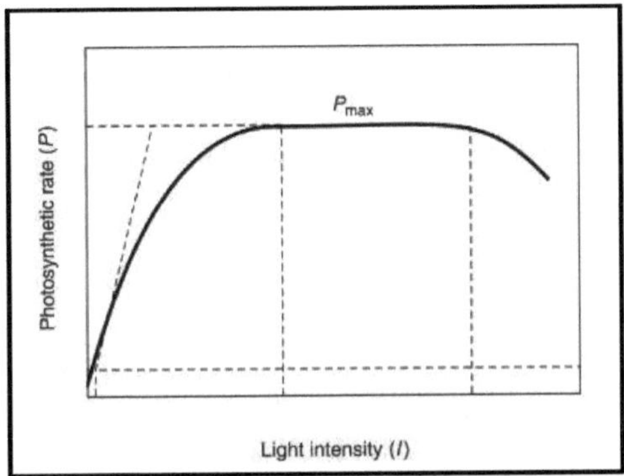

Figure 13: Spirulina photosynthesis rate as a function of light intensity .[41]

The interaction between light and temperature on spirulina growth has been extensively studied. The effect of photo-inhibition is accentuated at low temperatures, resulting in low cell concentration and productivity. However, these studies were carried out under natural lighting, where temperature and light intensity vary according to seasonal climatic changes and the photoperiod of the year.

When grown in darkness or at light intensities below 1000 lux, algae cultures produced very little biomass. On the contrary, a large amount of biomass was produced at higher light intensities of 1,500 to 3,500 lux. Soni *et al.* reported that at a light intensity of 2,500 lux, the best growth rates were achieved between 17° C and 37° C. The best biomass growth concentrations were obtained at 32° C with 12.28 g/l. However, production and growth rates were significantly lower at temperatures above 35° C and below 25° C. This may be due to the effect of temperature and light on photo-inhibition. Consequently, temperatures between 25° C and 35° C were optimal for spirulina cultivation in bioreactors**[42]**

2.5.2. Temperature

The most important physical factor influencing spirulina growth is temperature. Spirulina thrives best in water that reaches 38° C during the day

Above 43° C, the water is too hot and can be fatal for spirulina. On the other hand, below this temperature, the rate of multiplication decreases proportionally with temperature; at 20° C, growth virtually stops. The temperature of the culture medium must therefore be within this range .**[43]**

There is a specific light intensity for each temperature, which enables maximum photosynthesis activity to be achieved. Thus, the optimum temperature increases with light intensity. There is also an ideal temperature for maximizing biomass production. In addition, temperature variation influences cell composition: a drop in temperature increases the degree of lipid unsaturation, while a rise in temperature increases the concentration of oxygen free radicals and pigments .**[44]**

2.5.3. The pH

The optimum pH of a new culture medium depends on its use.

The pH must be at least 9 to start a new crop. If the pH is too low, the spirulina will precipitate to the bottom, indicating difficulties in starting the culture. On the other hand, if the medium is intended to supplement an existing culture, a pH close to 8 is acceptable. The addition of sodium bicarbonate helps maintain the high pH of the culture**[43]**

A pH increase of 0.1 units per day within a pH range of 10 to 10.6 is considered a positive indicator of crop growth. This increase occurs under these conditions: alkalinity of 0.1 N, spirulina concentration close to 0.4 g/l, liquid level around 20 cm, no carbon supplementation, no mineral deficiencies and high temperatures and sunshine. .**[28]**

A drop in pH can be caused by the presence of organic matter in the crop. This is due to the oxidation and release of CO_2.

To ensure that photosynthesis is taking place, you can observe the release of oxygen at the surface of the tank in the absence of any agitation .**[42]**

2.5.4. Carbon

Inorganic carbon is necessary for microalgae photosynthesis. Bicarbonate or CO_2 can be introduced by enriching the air supply. During photosynthesis, microalgae consume CO_2 solubilized in water. Depending on pH, the latter can exist in several states.

Focusing on reaction kinetics, the reaction that releases CO_2 is slower than the one involving bicarbonate (the protagonist), which occurs instantaneously.

Carbon dioxide is the predominant form of carbon at pH below 4.4. At pH 6.4, there are equal amounts of carbon dioxide and bicarbonate ions. The latter are equivalent to carbonate ions at pH 10.4.

Bicarbonate ions dominate at pH levels between 8.3 and 9.5, and above pH 12.3, carbonate ions dominate.

It takes 1.8 kg of carbon dioxide to produce 1 kg of biomass. As carbon dioxide is expensive, an alternative is to use plant effluents from combustion processes, which are available in large quantities and contribute to climate change.

This spirulina-based carbon sequestration technique was considered the most promising means of biological CO_2 sequestration for highly efficient photosynthesis and easy integration with other techniques**[45]** . Pre-treatment is sometimes required to concentrate the CO_2 and remove substances harmful to crops.**[29]**

2.5.5. Oxygen concentration

During phototrophic growth, microalgae generate oxygen (O_2) and absorb carbon dioxide (CO_2). The oxygen released can easily reach high concentrations in photobioreactors, and this can have a negative effect on biomass productivity by inhibiting microalgal cell growth. The main processes that can occur at high dissolved oxygen concentrations are generally attributed to photo-respiration and photo-inhibition. The latter occurs when microalgae are subjected to high light intensity levels over a long period, and leads to the generation of reactive oxygen species that can damage cellular components. Excessive concentrations of dissolved oxygen could be avoided by efficient air stripping to remove oxygen from the culture system. However, particular attention must be paid to maintaining a sufficiently high concentration of dissolved carbon in the culture medium, usually by simultaneously injecting CO_2. This dissolved carbon can thus reduce the negative impact of O_2-dependent photorespiration activity on the photosynthetic growth of microalgae .**[46]**

2.5.6. Nutritional requirements

To guarantee growth, the growing medium must contain the three main elementspotassium, phosphorus and nitrogen.

If calcium, magnesium and sulfur are not supplied in sufficient quantities by fertilizers, salt and water, supplementation is necessary**[47]**

Spirulina prefers ammonia and urea as sources of nitrogen. However, these substances become toxic above a certain concentration. For this reason, we often opt for nitrate, which can be added in high concentrations without danger to the crop, and thus constitutes a nitrogen reserve

Phosphorus can be introduced via monoammonium phosphate ($NH_4H_2PO_4$) or any other soluble orthophosphate. In some microalgae, phosphorus deficiency, like nitrogen deficiency, can manifest itself as pigment accumulations, but with less impact .**[28]**

Limiting nutrients, particularly nitrogen, is often an effective way of increasing specific target components in cells. Under nitrogen-stressed conditions, spirulina has the capacity to accumulate a significant proportion of lipids or carbohydrates. However, its growth rate decreases significantly with nitrogen limitation, which causes an overall decrease in biomass production and yield of desirable cellular components .**[48]**

2.5.7. Exopolysaccharide

Spirulina produces only exopolysaccharide (EPS) in the event of nitrogen deficiency. A sheath of EPS forms on the outer surface of spirulina when the concentration of EPS in the medium increases**[49]** . EPS clusters can slow down filtration by clogging the filters. The sieve retains bulky aggregates. At low pH and high light, normal EPS production is around 30% of that of spirulina.

A dose of 3 to 15 ppm ammonium, a pH above 10.2 and daily brushing of the pond bottom and walls can remedy this problem. In addition, the addition of calcium ions causes the precipitation of calcium carbonate and the elimination of EPS by flocculation .**[28]**

2.5.8. Mix

Mixing can be continuous or discontinuous (depending on the species). Its key roles are to prevent sedimentation and the formation of a gas or nutrient gradient, to reduce photo-limitation and photo-inhibition through homogeneous exposure of cells to the light gradient, to reduce the concentration of dissolved oxygen, and to promote the exchange of nutrients and metabolites within the culture**[29]**

Stirring with a cell-friendly electric agitator (paddle wheel, propeller, air bubbler, etc.) can be continuous, but 15-minute stops per hour are preferred. Continuous agitation with aquarium or vortex pumps is possible for wavy strains and some resistant spiral strains. Spiral strains are best agitated for only 15 to 30 minutes per hour. .**[28]**

2.5.9. Change in biomass as a function of initial concentration

Biomass concentration is one of the key parameters for system monitoring and design, and for optimizing growth rate and crop productivity .**[47]**

Figure 14 below shows spirulina growth as a function of initial concentration. Scissiparity (Spirulina's mode of reproduction) explains constant evolution between the curves for concentrations above 0.2 g/l. At high initial concentrations, spirulina multiplication is accompanied by rapid consumption of nutrients in the environment. This is followed by a depletion of resources, followed by a slowdown and then a cessation of growth**[50]**

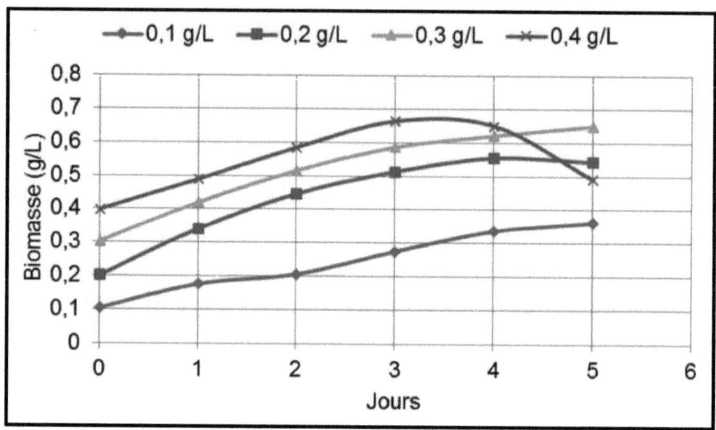

Figure 14: Evolution of biomass as a function of initial concentration[50]

Figure 15 shows a linear decrease in growth rate with increasing initial concentration: low growth rates are correlated with high initial concentrations. However, we note a high biomass productivity between 0.1 and 0.2 g/l, followed by a drop in biomass productivity between 0.2 and 0.4 g/l. These two curves lead us to adopt an optimum initial biomass concentration of 0.18 g/l.

However, the different productivities show a low mean deviation (4.29 mg/l/d). Thus, most appropriate initial inoculum concentration is the lowest: 0.05 g/l. In the same sense, high initial concentrations do not generate any significant difference in biomass production, which justifies their non-usefulness**[50]**

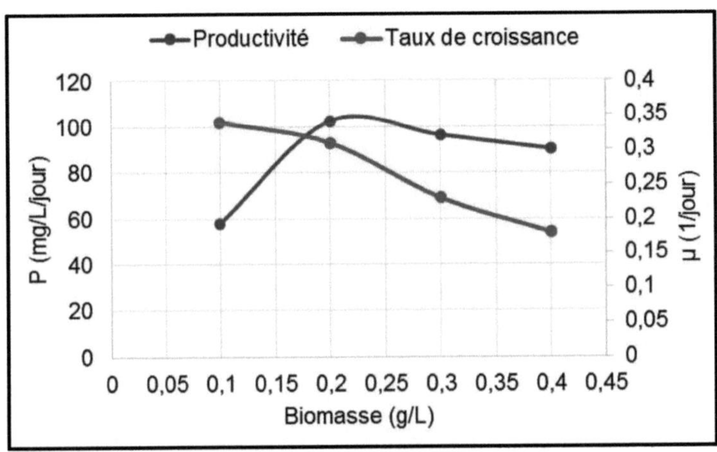

Figure 15: Evolution of productivity and growth rate as a function of initial biomass concentration[50]

3. QUALITY CONTROL

3.1.Description

Naturally, spirulina, which is blue-green in color, grows in lakes containing large quantities of organic matter and soda floating freely in salt water,**[51]** in the inter-tropical belt. Spirulina is harvested when it forms a green supernatant carried along by air currents on the surface of the water. It is then dried on sand to obtain a dehydrated form .**[52]**

There are around 2,000 species of Cyanobacteria, of which only 36 are edible. The main species currently on the market is *Spirulina platensis*. In France, the Agence nationale de sécurité de l'alimentation, de l'environnement et du travail (ANSES) has included only three spirulina species in its list of plants, other than mushrooms, authorized for use in food supplements. These are *S. major*, *S. platensis* and *S. maxima***[53]**

Industrially, spirulina extract is obtained by aqueous extraction of the biomass. The main pigments are two phycobiliproteins, C-phycocyanin and allophycocyanin .**[13]**

Phycocyanins, spirulina's main active ingredients, are pigments with an intense blue color and red fluorescence. Compared to chlorophyll, phycocyanins are less sensitive to photo-destruction, so their color becomes dominant as the chlorophyll green fades. On the other hand, when dried spirulina is rehydrated, phycocyanins quickly give the mixture an intense blue color: spirulina cells burst, releasing highly water-soluble proteins, while chlorophyll remains trapped in the cellular debris .**[5]**

One aspect of high-quality spirulina production is having a product with consistent chemical and physical properties**[38]**

3.2.Purity test

According to the residue monograph prepared in 2018 by the meeting of the Joint Expert Committee on Food Additives of the Food and Agriculture

Organization of the United Nations (FAO) and the World Health Organization (WHO), quality control must include a purity test consisting of the search for microcystins and a color test

3.2.1. Microcystins

Microcystins are hepatotoxic cyanotoxins. They are cyclic heptapeptides. They cause hepatic cytolysis, digestive disorders and liver failure on acute exposure, and hepatocarcinoma on chronic exposure. They can also cause kidney failure and neurological disorders. In 2003, the WHO defined a tolerable daily intake of 0.04 µg/kg/d for chronic exposure .**[54]**

An *enzyme-linked immunosorbent assay* (ELISA) is used to determine microcystins. Dry a suitable quantity of spirulina extract. Homogenize 3 g of the dried material in 20 ml of a methanol/water mixture (75:25, v/v) for 20 minutes. Centrifuge the resulting suspension at 4500 rpm for 10 minutes. Transfer the supernatant to a glass vial. Add 10 ml of methanol/water reagent to the homogenizer and homogenize the residue for 30 seconds. Centrifuge the resulting suspension at 4500 rpm for 10 minutes. Combine supernatants and dilute with water to the concentration specified by the ELISA kit manufacturer

In the *"Dietary Supplements Compendium"* the American Pharmacopoeia, a monograph devoted to *Arthrospira platensis* specifies a maximum microcystin content of 0.5 mg/kg by ELISA**[54]**

Spirulina companies such as *Earthrise* Farms have already developed methods for determining these toxins, and in fact certify that every batch of their product is toxin-free. Spirulina does not normally contain microcystins, but contamination of outdoor cultures by other cyanobacteria is possible .**[55]**

On the other hand, the ANSES in 2014, not clarify whether microcystins are substances to be controlled in spirulina-based dietary supplements .**[54]**

3.2.2. Staining test

This test is based on the absorbance of a buffered solution at 618 nm

Transfer 330 mg spirulina extract to a 100-ml volumetric flask and dilute to 100 ml with water. Transfer 10 ml of the solution into another 100 ml volumetric flask and dilute to 100 ml with sodium phosphate buffer (100 mM, pH= 6). Determine the absorbance of the solution in a 1 cm cell at 618 nm with an appropriate spectrophotometer, using sodium phosphate buffer (100 mM, pH= 6) as a reference.

Calculate the color value of spirulina extract as follows:

Color value = absorbance x 100 / weight of spirulina extract taken (g)

3.3.Microbial contamination

A potential problem with open-tank spirulina production is that the water may be contaminated with pathogenic organisms. Handling of the product during processing can also lead to microbial contamination. The final microbial load of the product therefore depends on the quality of handling with which the culture and product are treated at the various stages of production. Only good manufacturing practices and direct analysis of microbial flora and concentration can guarantee product safety. The final product must meet the microbiological standards set by the various national and international standards detailed in **table IX**. Total germ and total and faecal coliform counts are used in the food industry to monitor and inspect the handling of food products during processing. Analysis of hundreds of spirulina samples from commercial farms in Thailand, Japan and Mexico show that coliforms are rarely present, indicating good sanitary conditions for growth, harvesting, drying and packaging**[38]**

Table IX: Microbiological standards for spirulina[7]

	"American Herbal Products Association	**European Pharmacopoeia**	**Pharmacopoeia Japanese**
Total germs	10.000.000 IU/g	100,000 IU/g	<100,000 IU/g
Total coliforms	10.000 IU/g	no data	no data
Faecal coliforms	no data	no data	no data
Salmonella	Absent in 10g	Absent in 10g	Absent
Escherichia coli	Absent in 1g	Absent in 1g	Absent
Enterobacteriaceae	no data	1000 IU/g	1.000 IU/g
Staphylococcus	no data	Absent in 1g	no data
fragments	no data	Absent in 1g	no data
Rodent hair	no data	Absent in 1g	no data
	"World Heath Association **WHO**	*"National Nutritional Food Association*	*"Health Canada Compendium of Monographs*
Total germs	100,000 IU/g	50,000 IU/g	100,000 IU/g
Total coliforms	no data	10 IU/g	no data
Faecal coliforms	no data	Absent	no data
Salmonella	Absent	IU/g	Absent
Escherichia coli	10 IU/g	Absent	Absent
Enterobacteriaceae	1.000 IU/g	no data	no data
Staphylococcus	no data	most probable number(MPN)<10	<100 IU/g
fragments	no data	no data	no data
Rodent hair	no data	no data	no data

3.4.Heavy metal contamination

As in other agricultural products, lead, arsenic, mercury and cadmium are potential contaminants, as they are components of industrial pollution and are found in trace amounts in certain agricultural fertilizers. Some microalgae are known to be efficient accumulators of heavy metals. The production of high-quality spirulina therefore requires the use of high-quality nutrients and careful, regular analysis of heavy metals in the culture medium and in the product according to international standards illustrated in **Table X**. This is particularly important in situations where food-grade spirulina is to be produced from open ponds or natural lakes. The soil in some regions may have a high content of heavy metals, which can easily be accumulated by the algae.

Table X: Some examples of regulatory standards for heavy metals in dietary supplements and foods[56]

	***"Food and Drug Administration* FDA**	***Health Canada***	**WHO**	**European Union**
Arsenic	No data	<0.14 µ/d	2 µ/d	No data
Cadmium	55 µ/d	<0.09 µ/d	1 µ/d	<1 µ/d
lead	25 µ/d	<0.29 µ/d	3.6 µ/d	<3.6 µ/d
Mercure	1 ppm	<0.29	0.23 µ/d	0.23 µ/d

3.5.Pesticides

No pesticides or herbicides should be used during spirulina cultivation. Even if the high pH of the environment hinders the persistence of pesticides, it is imperative to periodically monitor the presence of pesticides in the product (spring water, growing water, etc.) .**[38]**

The use of pesticides is an obsolete practice, given the virtual absence of pests and parasites in spirulina crops. Spirulina is highly sensitive to most herbicides, whether they affect nitrogen metabolism and the photosynthetic system, such as triazines, or lipid synthesis, such as pyridazinones.

Taken together, these data no doubt explain the absence in the literature of any significant cases of pesticide contamination of spirulina**[5]**

3.6.Foreign materials

The material is brought in by insects, rodents, binders or other animal contamination. The main components of foreign matter in food products are insect fragments and rodent hair. A standardized analytical method is used to count insect fragments. Although sample preparation and counting are highly standardized, it is preferable to select a batch for the identification process. Distinguishing between insect parts and plant parts is often tricky, leading to an overestimation of these fragments.

The new method quantifies the biomass of insect fragments in microalgae products using an ELISA test. This new method is an improvement on the standard method, which records the number of insect fragments independently of large differences in insect fragment size.

The presence of rodent hair is considered an indicator of potential contamination. It is very rare to observe rodent hair when daily checks are carried out**[38]**

3.7.Cyanobacterial toxins

The techniques used to detect cyanobacteria are an ELISA test (highly sensitive) and a phosphatase inhibition test for the detection of specific toxins. These methods enable the detection, monitoring and control of cyanotoxins to guarantee product quality**[38]**

It has been confirmed that certain toxins secreted by cyanobacteria have an effect on the nervous system or liver. In the case of cultivated spirulina, no such toxins have been identified.

However, in Chad, algae such as *Mycrocystis aeruginosa* and *Anabaenopsis circularis* periodically invade lakes containing spirulina. These seasonal contaminations reflect changes in the composition of the environment, such as changes in pH due to rainfall or a sharp drop in salinity. These changes can be controlled by artificial cultivation**[5]**

3.8.Polycyclic aromatic hydrocarbons

Incomplete combustion of organic matter produces polycyclic aromatic hydrocarbons (PAHs). During the drying process, spirulina becomes contaminated with these PAHs. According to European Union standards, levels of benzo(a)pyrene and ΣHAP4 (benzo(b)fluoranthene, benzo(k)fluorathene, benzo(ghi)perylene and indeno(1,2,3-cd)pyrene, which are possible human carcinogens) must not exceed 10 μg / kg and 50 μg / kg, respectively .**[57]**

4. FOOD SUPPLEMENTS AND CLAIMS

4.1.Definitions

In 2002, the European Commission defined food supplements as "foodstuffs the purpose of which is to supplement the body's own diet".
normal diet and which constitute a concentrated source of nutrients or other substances having a nutritional or physiological effect alone or in combination...".
A claim is any assertion that states, suggests or implies that a food has particular properties.
We define 2 types of claims

- Nutritional claim: provides information on the nutrient or energy content of a foodstuff.
- Health claim: indicates, suggests or implies the existence of a relationship between a nutrient or food and a state of health .**[58]**

4.2.Legislative and regulatory developments for spirulina

Before 2002, there was no strict definition of a dietary supplement.
Spirulina was subject to food regulations, as it was classified as a foodstuff.
In 2011, spirulina was classified as a safe ingredient in dietary supplements. It is the only blue microalgae recognized as GRAS**[59]** "*Generally Recognized As Safe*" by the FDA**[60]** and the US Pharmacopoeia Committee, which reviewed dietary supplements containing spirulina, to determine whether it should be admitted as a quality monograph in the US Pharmacopoeia and National Formulary. Following this evaluation, a monograph for *Arthrospira platensis* is now available in the USP .**[61]**
Spirulina extracts are listed by the Codex Alimentarius as food additives, classified as colorants. In China, Japan, Korea and the USA, spirulina is also approved as a food additive, used as a food coloring agent.

Specifications for maximum concentration limits in foodstuffs are in the range of 0.5 to 2% m/m for spirulina extracts or concentrates .**[54]**
Spirulina is classified as a foodstuff in France and is recognized as a food by the FAO. It is not considered a medicinal product in France or Europe.
Spirulina has not been evaluated by the Food *Safety* Authority (EFSA), has no corresponding data from the Agence nationale de sécurité du médicament (ANSM) or the European *Medicines* Agency EMA), and is not listed in the French Pharmacopoeia.
Food supplements, which for a long time had no legislative framework of their own, have been the subject of numerous laws in recent years to regulate their use. They are also subject to strict regulations concerning the claims they make. Manufacturers are required to provide a high level of proof, and many insufficiently documented claims have been rejected. The aim of this new legislative framework is to guarantee French and European consumers a high level of safety when consuming food supplements**[62]**

5. EMPLOYMENT S

5.1.Spirulina for human use

5.1.1. Nutritional claims

According to the monograph in *Heath Canada*, the use of spirulina as a source of protein, β-carotene and iron is acceptable. These claims are detailed in **Tables XI** and **XII**.

Furthermore, *Heath Canada* and ANSES indicate that spirulina cannot be considered a reliable source of vitamin B12 for individuals who do not consume animal products, as the majority of vitamin B_{12} present in spirulina is not bioactive. .**[54]**

5.1.1.1. Claims based on the protein component

In terms of composition, spirulina's protein content is the most interesting. **Table XI** shows the recommended daily doses of algal protein for different age groups.

Table XI: Daily doses of algal protein (no minimum dose of spirulina required)

Sub-population(s)		Minimum dose of algal protein (g/day)	Maximum dose seaweed and spirulina protein (g/day)
Children	2 to 4 years	0,6	1
	5 to 9 years	0,9	2
	10 to 11 years	1,5	4
Teenagers	12 to 14 years	1,5	4
	15 to 17 years	2,6	8
Adults	18 and over	2,6	8

5.1.1.2. Claims based on the constituents beta-carotene or iron

Table XII shows recommended daily doses for different age groups.

Table XII: Daily doses of beta-carotene and iron (no minimum spirulina dose required)

Sub-population(s)		Beta-carotene		Iron		Maximum spirulina dose (g/day)
		Min (mcg/day)	Max (mcg/day)	Min (mg/day)	Max (mg/day)	
Children	2 to 3 years	180	3600	0,6	40	1
	4 years	180	5400	0,6	40	1
	5 to 8 years	180	5400	0,6	40	2
	9 years old	180	10200	0,6	40	2
	10 to 11 years	180	10200	0,6	40	4
Teenagers	12 to 13 years	180	10200	0,6	40	4
	14 years old	390	16800	1,4	45	4
	15 to 17 years	390	16800	1,4	45	8
Adults	18 years old	390	16800	1,4	45	8
	19 and over	390	18000	1,4	45	8

5.1.2. Health claims

Spirulina has numerous health claims. Those listed in **Table XIII** are still pending, according to the Syndicat National des Compléments Alimentaires.

Table XIII: Health applications and claims according to the Syndicat Nationale des Compléments Alimentaires in 2017 .[54]

Application	Pending claims	Dosages
Antioxidant	Helps protect against oxidative stress.	2 to 3g/ day
Tonic	Helps boost energy and vitality Helps combat fatigue, improves vitality and energy.	2g/d
Natural decences	Boosts the immune system Phycocyanin is a powerful stimulant of natural defenses Strengthens the body's resistance	2 to 3g/day
moderator	Control weight by preventing starch degradation	1.8 g/d

As shown in **Table XIV**, *"Health Canada"* presents only allergic rhinitis/antioxidant as a health claim. 0note that no minimum dose of spirulina is set for an antioxidant effect; however, it is important to respect the maximum recommended dose .**[54]**

Table XIV: Daily doses of spirulina for allergic rhinitis.

Sub-population(s)		Minimum dose (g/day)	Maximum dose (g/d)
Child	2 to 4 years	0,3	1
	5 to 9 years	0,5	2
	10 to 11 years	1	4
teenagers	12 to 14 years	1	4
	15 to 17 years	2	8
Adults	18 and over	2	8

5.2.Usage animal

Spirulina is used as a food supplement for very specific effects in aquariums, aquaculture and food processing .**[63]**

Spirulina can promote growth and fertility in several animal species. Studies on a species of tropical freshwater fish, *Xiphophorus helleri*, and on the fleshy shrimp *Fenneropenaeus chinensis* have demonstrated the beneficial effects of *Spirulina platensis* in this area.

Thanks to its pigments, spirulina is also used to enhance the coloration of ornamental fish, and to improve the pigmentation of shrimp and fish in aquaculture.

It can, however, boost the immune system. Spirulina is added to the pelleted feed of farmed fish, which are more susceptible to bacterial and viral infections than wild fish .**[64]**

In the food industry, thanks to its carotenoids, Spirulina is used to make eggs and chicken meat more attractive to consumers.

Finally, spirulina is used to improve the performance of racehorses and breeding bulls .**[8]**

All these combined uses converge towards optimized weight control and improved growth, feed conversion and reproductive performance .**[65]**

5.3.Industrial use

5.3.1. Natural colorant

Pigments, more commonly known as "colorants", are substances that add color to foods and other products. Synthetic colorants are banned in many countries. On the other hand, natural colorants produced by microorganisms have gained a foothold on the market. Pigments are mainly used in foods, pharmaceutical products, cosmetics, ice cream, candies, soft drinks and dairy products.

The main pigments present in spirulina are chlorophylls, carotenoids and phycobiliproteins. Typical phycobilin pigments include C-phycocyanin and allophycocyanin .**[65]**
It is very difficult to isolate stable natural blue dyes that match the shade of brilliant blue. The closest alternative to brilliant blue has been isolated from spirulina biomass. The blue color (λ_{max} = 618 nm) comes from phycocyanin .**[19]**

5.3.2. Pollution control

One of the most recent solutions for minimizing CO_2 emissions into the atmosphere is the biofixation of CO(2) by spirulina (direct injection into photobioreactors). This is an alternative for the sustainable use of coal. What's more, the biomass obtained can be used to produce biotechnological products such as biofuels: biodiesel, bioethanol, etc. .**[66]**
Spirulina is also attracting attention for its valuable potential to bioaccumulate heavy metals**[67]**lead, mercury, arsenic, cadmium and chromium. These metals are carcinogenic and toxic even at trace levels**[68]** . In this context, both living cells and non-living biomass can be used. Spirulina can also be used to recover precious metal ions, such as thallium, silver and gold .**[69]**
Spirulina's ability to survive under conditions of salt stress has shed light on its potential use in the field of wastewater exploitation. This water can be used as a culture medium, helping to reduce the cost of biomass production .**[70]**

5.3.3. Renewable energy source

The use of fuels such as oil and coal poses a considerable threat in terms of pollution of the terrestrial and marine environment and deterioration of air quality. Spirulina is proving to be a new source of fuels (known as biofuels) .**[71]**
Spirulina can be used to produce bioethanol, biomethane**[72]** and biohydrogen**[66]** as its biomass has a high carbohydrate and lipid content**[73]** . Fuel production from spirulina can be improved by selecting strains with high

oil content, improving growth rates**[71]** and developing efficient oil extraction and harvesting techniques .**[74]**

Bioethanol (identical to ethanol) has a high potential to reduce emissions, particularly particulate emissions .**[75]**

Biochemical and thermochemical conversion,**[76]** such as transesterification, pyrolysis**[77]** , gasification, hydrothermal liquefaction**[78]** and enzymatic lysis**[79]** , can be used to convert biomass feedstock into biofuels.

Spirulina has been used not only for biofuels, but also in electrochemical materials, food science and other fields .**[80]**

6. TOXICITY, ADVERSE EFFECTS AND PRECAUTIONS

Most studies have focused on the beneficial effects of spirulina. A minority focused on adverse effects attributed to spirulina. Three clinical studies, dozens of reports from pharmacovigilance centers and three clinical cases reported adverse effects of a digestive, hepatic or dermatological nature, as well as hematological, renal and electrolytic disorders.

Randomized, placebo-controlled clinical trials were conducted by Branger *et al* (2003), Yamani *et al* (2009) and Marcel *et al* (2011). Only the latter reported serious adverse events in pulmonary tuberculosis.

The three clinical case studies are by Mazokopakis *et al* (2008), Kraigher *et al* (2008) and Iwassa *et al* (2002). All three reported rhabdomyolysis, dermatitis and hepatotoxicity respectively .**[81]**

Mazokopakis *et al.* reported a case of acute rhabdomyolysis in a 28-year-old man who had been taking spirulina tablets as a dietary supplement (at an intake of 3g/day, recommended by the manufacturer) for one month prior to the onset of symptoms. The patient was not taking any other medication, and reportedly did not consume alcohol or illicit drugs. Biological tests suggested rhabdomyolysis, marked by elevated concentrations of creatinine kinase and other muscle enzymes such as myoglobin, alanine aminotransferase, aspartate aminotransferase, lactate dehydrogenase and aldolase. The patient was hydrated for 4 days, then discharged from hospital. A week later, symptoms disappeared and laboratory results were normal.

Iwasa *et al.* reported elevated liver enzyme concentrations in a 52-year-old Japanese man who had used a spirulina-based product for 5 weeks. The patient had a history of hypertension, hyperlipidemia and type 2 diabetes, and had been taking simvastatin and amlodipine for 7 months. Unfortunately, the article did not discuss the well-documented possibility that a statin such as simvastatin could cause liver damage. The report concluded that the adverse effect may have been amputated to spirulina, as the patient's liver enzyme concentrations improved after its withdrawal. However, all the patient's medications were stopped simultaneously, so other explanations for the drop in liver enzyme concentrations cannot be ruled out .**[61]**

The United States Pharmacopeia, with the aim establishing a monograph for spirulina, has collected reports of adverse reactions to spirulina from pharmacovigilance centers worldwide since 1996 and over a 12-year period. A total of 31 reports were examined. The *MedWatch* report from the USA reported 11 cases of adverse reactions, compared with 8 cases in *The Canada Vigilance Program* and 2 cases in an Australian report. The WHO Pharmacovigilance Center reported 10 cases. Spirulina has been shown to be responsible for these adverse reactions. Classifying adverse reactions by pathological area in **Table XV**, those related to the hepatic system come in first place, followed by dermatological and digestive effects .**[81]**

Table XV: Summary of adverse reactions to spirulina reported to pharmacovigilance centers[81]

Patholog	Number of declarations	Percentages
Hepatic	12	34.30
dermatological	7	20
digestive	6	17.14
Central nervous system	3	8.57
hematological	3	8.57
nephrology	1	2.85
electrolytic	3	8.57

Consumers and patients need to be aware of the importance of sourcing spirulina via a properly authenticated circuit. They should inform their doctors or pharmacists about the use of spirulina-based dietary supplements, particularly in the event of undesirable side effects. Specific and fragile populations (the elderly, chronically ill, pregnant women and children) will also be informed and warned .**[82]**

In 2010, Health Canada also reported two cases of adverse reactions

- An elderly woman had used six products concomitantly, including one containing spirulina, and experienced abdominal pain accompanied by nausea and hyperamylasemia. Her condition improved within an unrecorded time.
- An individual of unknown age and sex, who had consumed spirulina and another product concomitantly, also presented with digestive problems. The outcome is unknown.

Assessing the characteristics of spirulina and the spectrum of adverse effects reported, ANSES advises against the consumption of these dietary supplements "in individuals with phenylketonuria, allergic conditions or muscular or hepatic vulnerability" .**[54]**

CONCLUSION

Spirulina's nutritional and therapeutic properties, its exceptional macro- and micronutrient composition and its many applications make it a rich food source that deserves special attention in our country, where climatic conditions are considered favorable for cultivation and production.

It contains molecules of pharmaceutical interest, such as polyphenolic compounds, phycocyanin and β-carotene. These substances have been the subject of numerous recent scientific publications, and could in future form part of curative and preventive treatments for serious diseases.

Promoting spirulina production in Tunisia could have a positive impact on the economy. This would encourage job creation and the development of small businesses and startups.

Studies carried out on spirulina suggest that it is safe in healthy subjects, but it remains a little-known product (with acceptability yet to be assessed) and poorly controlled in Tunisia. Microbiological control and the detection of accidental contamination, as well as the evaluation of chemical and physical characteristics to ensure a high-quality product that meets the requirements of various international standards, commitments to consumers.

Unfortunately, these requirements are not always met, given the shortcomings of the legislative framework for dietary supplements in Tunisia.

This legal vacuum has led to the development of a growing number of food supplements promising vitality, beauty and well-being, often without any real scientific validation, putting consumers' health at risk.

REFERENCES

1. Vaz BS, Moreira JB, Morais MG, Costa JA. Microalgae as a new source of bioactive compounds in food supplements. Curr Opin Food Sci. 2016;7:73-7.
2. Balti R, Zayoud N, Hubert F, Beaulieu L, Massé A. Fractionation of Arthrospira platensis (Spirulina) water soluble proteins by membrane diafiltration. Sep Purif Technol. 2021;256:1-10.
3. Finamore A, Palmery M, Bensehaila S, Peluso I. Antioxidant, immunomodulating, and microbial-modulating activities of the sustainable and ecofriendly spirulina. Oxid Med Cell Longev. 2017;2017:1-14.
4. Soni RA, Sudhakar K, Rana RS. Spirulina - from growth to nutritional product: A review. Trends Food Sci Technol. 2017;69:157-71.
5. Vicat JP, Doumnang Mbaigane JC, Bellion Y. Major and trace element contents of spirulina (Arthrospira platensis) from France, Chad, Togo, Niger, Mali, Burkina-Faso and Central African Republic. C R Biol. 2014;337(1):44-52.
6. Lupatini AL, Colla LM, Canan C, Colla E. Potential application of microalga Spirulina platensis as a protein source: Potential application of microalga Spirulina platensis as a protein source. J Sci Food Agric. 2017;97(3):724-32.
7. Carcea M, Sorto M, Batello C, Narducci V, Aguzzi A, Azzini E, et al. Nutritional characterization of traditional and improved dihé, alimentary blue-green algae from the lake Chad region in Africa. LWT - Food Sci Technol. 2015;62(1):753-63.

8. Charpy L. Can Spirulina be an asset for health and development in Africa?[Online]. 2008 [Accessed April 18, 2021]. Available at: http://www.plancton-du-monde.org/fileadmin/ documents/IRD_spiruine_atout_developpement_afrique.pdf
9. Nowicka-Krawczyk P, Mühlsteinová R, Hauer T. Detailed characterization of the Arthrospira type species separating commercially grown taxa into the new genus Limnospira (Cyanobacteria). Sci Rep. 2019;9(1):694.
10. Falquet J. Spirulina Aspects Nutritionnels [Online]. 2006 [Accessed April 18, 2021]. Available at: https://www.antenna.ch/wp-content/uploads/2017/04/AspNutr2006.pdf
11. Aiello G, Li Y, Boschin G, Bollati C, Arnoldi A, Lammi C. Chemical and biological characterization of spirulina protein hydrolysates: Focus on ACE and DPP-IV activities modulation. J Funct Foods. 2019;63:1-8.
12. Marfaing H. Nutritional qualities of algae, their present and future on the food scene. Cah Nutr Diet. 2017;52(5):257-68.
13. Manirafasha E, Murwanashyaka T, Ndikubwimana T, Rashid Ahmed N, Liu J, Lu Y, et al. Enhancement of cell growth and phycocyanin production in Arthrospira (Spirulina) platensis by metabolic stress and nitrate fed-batch. Bioresour Technol. 2018;255:293-301.
14. Li TT, Tong AJ, Liu YY, Huang ZR, Wan XZ, Pan YY, et al. Polyunsaturated fatty acids from microalgae Spirulina platensis modulates lipid metabolism disorders and gut microbiota in high-fat diet rats. Food Chem Toxicol. 2019;131:1-9.
15. Crampon C, Nikitine C, Zaier M, Lépine O, Tanzi CD, Vian MA, et al. Oil extraction from enriched Spirulina platensis microalgae using supercritical carbon dioxide. J Supercrit Fluids. 2017;119:289-96.

16. Alshuniaber MA, Krishnamoorthy R, AlQhtani WH. Antimicrobial activity of polyphenolic compounds from Spirulina against food-borne bacterial pathogens. Saudi J Biol Sci. 2021;28(1):459-64.

17. Christ-Ribeiro A, Graça CS, Kupski L, Badiale-Furlong E, de Souza-Soares LA. Cytotoxicity, antifungal and anti mycotoxins effects of phenolic compounds from fermented rice bran and Spirulina sp. Process Biochem. 2019;80:190-6.

18. Hsieh-Lo M, Castillo G, Ochoa-Becerra MA, Mojica L. Phycocyanin and phycoerythrin: Strategies to improve production yield and chemical stability. Algal Res. 2019;42:1-11.

19. Li Y, Zhang Z, Paciulli M, Abbaspourrad A. Extraction of phycocyanin-A natural blue colorant from dried spirulina biomass: Influence of processing parameters and extraction techniques. J Food Sci. 2020;85(3):727-35.

20. Girardin-Andréani C. Spirulina: blood system, immune system and cancer. Phytotherapie. 2005;3(4):158-61.

21. Wu Q, Liu L, Miron A, Klímová B, Wan D, Kuča K. The antioxidant, immunomodulatory, and anti-inflammatory activities of Spirulina: an overview. Arch Toxicol. 2016;90(8):1817-40.

22. Liu Q, Huang Y, Zhang R, Cai T, Cai Y. Medical application of Spirulina platensis derived C-Phycocyanin. Evid Based Complement Alternat Med. 2016;2016:1-14.

23. Rajasekar P, Palanisamy S, Anjali R, Vinosha M, Elakkiya M, Marudhupandi T, et al. Isolation and structural characterization of sulfated polysaccharide from Spirulina platensis and its bioactive potential: In

vitro antioxidant, antibacterial activity and Zebrafish growth and reproductive performance. Int J Biol Macromol. 2019;141:809-21.

24. Silva A, Magalhães WT, Moreira LM, Rocha MV, Bastos AK. Microwave-assisted extraction of polysaccharides from Arthrospira (Spirulina) platensis using the concept of green chemistry. Algal Res. 2018;35:178-84.

25. Ugwu CU, Aoyagi H, Uchiyama H. Photobioreactors for mass cultivation of algae. Bioresour Technol. 2008;99(10):4021-8.

26. Deamici KM, Santos LO, Costa JA. Magnetic field action on outdoor and indoor cultures of Spirulina: Evaluation of growth, medium consumption and protein profile. Bioresour Technol. 2018;249:168-74.

27. Efroymson RA, Pattullo MB, Mayes MA, Mathews TJ, Mandal S, Schoenung S. Exploring the sustainability and sealing mechanisms of unlined ponds for growing algae for fuel and other commodity-scale products. Renew Sustain Energy Rev. 2020;121:1-10.

28. Jourdan JP. Manual de culture artisanale de la spiruline [Online]. 2013 [Accessed April 18, 2021]. Available at: https://www.antenna.ch/wp-content/uploads/2017/04/Manuel_Cultivez_votre_spiruline_REVISION_2013.pdf

29. Lucchetti A. Modeling and design of a microalgae culture system [Thesis]. Paris: École Nationale Supérieure des Mines de Paris; 2014.

30. Sierra E, Acién FG, Fernández JM, García JL, González C, Molina E. Characterization of a flat plate photobioreactor for the production of microalgae. Chem Eng J. 2008;138:136-47.

31.Zhang Q, Wu X, Xue S, Liang K, Cong W. Study of hydrodynamic characteristics in tubular photobioreactors. Bioprocess Biosyst Eng. 2013;36(2):143-50.

32.Vree JH, Bosma R, Janssen M, Barbosa MJ, Wijffels RH. Comparison of four outdoor pilot-scale photobioreactors. Biotechnol Biofuels. 2015;8(1):1-12.

33.Duan Y, Shi F. Bioreactor design for algal growth as a sustainable energy source. In: Shi F, editor. Reactor and process design in sustainable energy technology. Amsterdam: Elsevier; 2014. p. 27-60.

34.Madkour FF, Kamil AE, Nasr HS. Production and nutritive value of Spirulina platensis in reduced cost media. Egypt J Aquat Res. 2012;38(1):51-7.

35.Nazari MT, Rigueto CV, Rempel A, Colla LM. Harvesting of Spirulina platensis using an eco-friendly fungal bioflocculant produced from agro-industrial by-products. Bioresour Technol. 2021;322:1-8.

36.Vonshak A. Strain selection of Spirulina suitable for mass production. In: Ragan MA, Bird CJ, editors. Twelfth international seaweed symposium. Dordrecht: Springer Netherlands; 1987. p. 75-7.

37.Niangoran NU. Optimization of spirulina cultivation in a controlled environment: lighting and biomass estimation [Thesis]. Toulouse: École Doctorale Génie électrique, électronique et télécommunications de Toulouse; 2017.

38.Jin SE, Lee SJ, Park CY. Mass-production and biomarker-based characterization of high-value Spirulina powder for nutritional supplements. Food Chem. 2020;325:1-6.

39.Fradinho P, Niccolai A, Soares R, Rodolfi L, Biondi N, Tredici MR, et al. Effect of Arthrospira platensis (spirulina) incorporation on the rheological and bioactive properties of gluten-free fresh pasta. Algal Res. 2020;45:1-12.

40. Ye C, Mu D, Horowitz N, Xue Z, Chen J, Xue M, et al. Life cycle assessment of industrial scale production of spirulina tablets. Algal Res. 2018;34:154-63.

41. Raeisossadati M, Moheimani NR, Parlevliet D. Luminescent solar concentrator panels for increasing the efficiency of mass microalgal production. Renew Sustain Energy Rev. 2019;101:47-59.

42. Soni RA, Sudhakar K, Rana RS. Comparative study on the growth performance of Spirulina platensis on modifying culture media. Energy Rep. 2019;5:327-36.

43. Pandey J, Pathak N, Tiwari A. Standardization of pH and light intensity for the biomass production of Spirulina platensis. J Algal Biomass Utln. 2010;1:93-102.

44. Yuan S, Hu J, Liu Z, Hong Y, Wang X. Modeling microalgae growth in continuous culture: Parameters analysis and temperature dependence. Energy. 2020;195:1-10.

45. Liu H, Chen H, Wang S, Liu Q, Li S, Song X, et al. Optimizing light distribution and controlling biomass concentration by continuously pre-harvesting Spirulina platensis for improving the microalgae production. Bioresour Technol. 2018;252:14-9.

46. Kazbar A, Cogne G, Urbain B, Marec H, Le-Gouic B, Tallec J, et al. Effect of dissolved oxygen concentration on microalgal culture in photobioreactors. Algal Res. 2019;39:1-49.

47. Su Y, Mennerich A, Urban B. A comparison of feasible methods for microalgal biomass determinations during tertiary wastewater treatment. Ecol Eng. 2016;94:532-6.

48. Li X, Li W, Zhai J, Wei H. Effect of nitrogen limitation on biochemical composition and photosynthetic performance for fed-batch mixotrophic cultivation of microalga Spirulina platensis. Bioresour Technol. 2018;263:555-61.

49. Sardar UR, Bhargavi E, Devi I, Bhunia B, Tiwari ON. Advances in exopolysaccharides based bioremediation of heavy metals in soil and water: A critical review. Carbohydr Polym. 2018;199:353-64.

50. Shi W, Li S, Li G, Wang W, Chen Q, Li Y, et al. Investigation of main factors affecting the growth rate of Spirulina. Optik. 2016;127(16):6688-94.

51. Czerwonka A, Kaławaj K, Sławińska-Brych A, Lemieszek MK, Bartnik M, Wojtanowski KK, et al. Anticancer effect of the water extract of a commercial Spirulina (Arthrospira platensis) product on the human lung cancer A549 cell line. Biomed Pharmacother. 2018;106:292-302.

52. Inrae. Lettre scientifique synadiet [Online]. 2017 [Accessed April 17, 2021]. Available from: https://www6.inrae.fr/cost-positive/content/download/3910/37144/version/1/file/LettreScientifiqueSynadiet%20n%C2%B02.pdf

53. Fleurence J, Levine IA. Antiallergic and allergic properties. In: Levine IA, Fleurence J, editors. Microalgae in health and disease prevention. Cambridge: Academic Press; 2018 . p. 307-15.

54. ANSES. Risks associated with the consumption of dietary supplements containing spirulina [Online]. 2017 [Accessed April 18, 2021]. Available at: https://www.anses.fr/fr/system/files/NUT2014SA0096.pdf
55. Shimamatsu H. Mass production of Spirulina, an edible microalga. Hydrobiologia. 2004;512:39-44.
56. Gershwin ME, Belay A. Spirulina in Human Nutrition and Health. CRC Press; 2007.
57. Muys M, Sui Y, Schwaiger B, Lesueur C, Vandenheuvel D, Vermeir P, et al. High variability in nutritional value and safety of commercially available Chlorella and Spirulina biomass indicates the need for smart production strategies. Bioresour Technol. 2019;275:247-57.
58. Cynober L. Food supplement, health food, medicine: Who's who? Or faust revisited. Cah Nutr Diet. 2008;43(1):15-21.
59. Verdasco-Martín CM, Díaz-Lozano A, Otero C. Advantageous enzyme selective extraction process of essential spirulina oil. Catal Today. 2020;346:121-31.
60. Lucas BF, Morais MG, Santos TD, Costa JA. Spirulina for snack enrichment: Nutritional, physical and sensory evaluations. Food Sci Technol. 2018;90:270-6.
61. Marles RJ, Barrett ML, Barnes J, Chavez ML, Gardiner P, Ko R, et al. United States pharmacopeia safety evaluation of Spirulina. Crit Rev Food Sci Nutr. 2011;51(7):593-604.
62. Pilorin T, Hébel P. Consumption of dietary supplements in France: consumer profile and contribution to nutritional balance. Cah Nutr Diet. 2012;47(3):147-55.

63.Jin SE, Lee SJ, Kim Y, Park CY. Spirulina powder as a feed supplement to enhance abalone growth. Aquac Rep. 2020;17:1-8.

64.Adel M, Yeganeh S, Dadar M, Sakai M, Dawood MA. Effects of dietary Spirulina platensis on growth performance, humoral and mucosal immune responses and disease resistance in juvenile great sturgeon (Huso huso Linnaeus, 1754). Fish Shellfish Immunol. 2016;56:436-44.

65.Costa JA, Freitas BC, Rosa GM, Moraes L, Morais MG, Mitchell BG. Operational and economic aspects of Spirulina-based biorefinery. Bioresour Technol. 2019;292:1-10.

66.Duarte JH, Morais EG, Radmann EM, Costa JA. Biological CO2 mitigation from coal power plant by Chlorella fusca and Spirulina sp. Bioresour Technol. 2017;234:472-5.

67.Choi YK, Choi TR, Gurav R, Bhatia SK, Park YL, Kim HJ, et al. Adsorption behavior of tetracycline onto Spirulina sp. (microalgae)-derived biochars produced at different temperatures. Sci Total Environ. 2020;710:1-11.

68.Cepoi L, Zinicovscaia I, Rudi L, Chiriac T, Miscu V, Djur S, et al. Growth and heavy metals accumulation by Spirulina platensis biomass from multicomponent copper containing synthetic effluents during repeated cultivation cycles. Ecol Eng. 2020;142:1-12.

69.Leong YK, Chang JS. Bioremediation of heavy metals using microalgae: Recent advances and mechanisms. Bioresour Technol. 2020;303:1-11.

70.Mata SN, Souza Santos T, Cardoso LG, Andrade BB, Duarte JH, Costa JA, et al. Spirulina sp. LEB 18 cultivation in a raceway-type bioreactor using wastewater from desalination process: Production of carbohydrate-rich biomass. Bioresour Technol. 2020;311:1-7.

71.Sharma YC, Singh V. Microalgal biodiesel: A possible solution for India's energy security. Renew Sustain Energy Rev. 2017;67:72-88.

72.Rempel A, Souza Sossella F, Margarites AC, Astolfi AL, Steinmetz RLR, Kunz A, et al. Bioethanol from Spirulina platensis biomass and the use of residuals to produce biomethane: An energy efficient approach. Bioresour Technol. 2019;288:1-8.

73.Luiza Astolfi A, Rempel A, Cavanhi VA, Alves M, Deamici KM, Colla LM, et al. Simultaneous saccharification and fermentation of Spirulina sp. and corn starch for the production of bioethanol and obtaining biopeptides with high antioxidant activity. Bioresour Technol. 2020;301:1-7.

74.Pohndorf RS, Camara ÁS, Larrosa AP, Pinheiro CP, Strieder MM, Pinto LA. Production of lipids from microalgae Spirulina sp.: Influence of drying, cell disruption and extraction methods. Biomass Bioenergy. 2016;93:25-32.

75.Rajak U, Nashine P, Nath Verma T. Numerical study on emission characteristics of a diesel engine fuelled with diesel-spirulina microalgae-ethanol blends at various operating conditions. Fuel. 2020;262:1-20.

76.Chen H, He Z, Zhang B, Feng H, Kandasamy S, Wang B. Effects of the aqueous phase recycling on bio-oil yield in hydrothermal liquefaction of Spirulina Platensis, α-cellulose, and lignin. Energy. 2019;179:1103-13.

77.Dai M, Yu Z, Fang S, Ma X. Behaviors, product characteristics and kinetics of catalytic co-pyrolysis spirulina and oil shale. Energy Convers Manag. 2019;192:1-10.

78.Kandasamy S, Zhang B, He Z, Chen H, Feng H, Wang Q, et al. Effect of low-temperature catalytic hydrothermal liquefaction of Spirulina platensis. Energy. 2020;190:1-12.

79. Zhang B, Feng H, He Z, Wang S, Chen H. Bio-oil production from hydrothermal liquefaction of ultrasonic pre-treated Spirulina platensis. Energy Convers Manag. 2018;159:204-12.

80. Xiao H, Zhai Y, Xie J, Wang T, Wang B, Li S, et al. Speciation and transformation of nitrogen for spirulina hydrothermal carbonization. Bioresour Technol. 2019;286:1-7.

81. Barry M, Ouedraogo M, Ouedraogo M, Sourabie S, Guissou I, Pierrick B, et al. Reporting adverse effects of spirulina in humans: a systematic review. Int J Biol Chem Sci. 2014;7(4):1568-78.

82. Crenn P. Benefits and risks of dietary supplements. Nutr Clin Métabolisme. 2020;34(3):201-6.

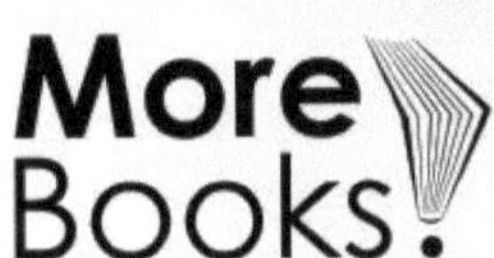

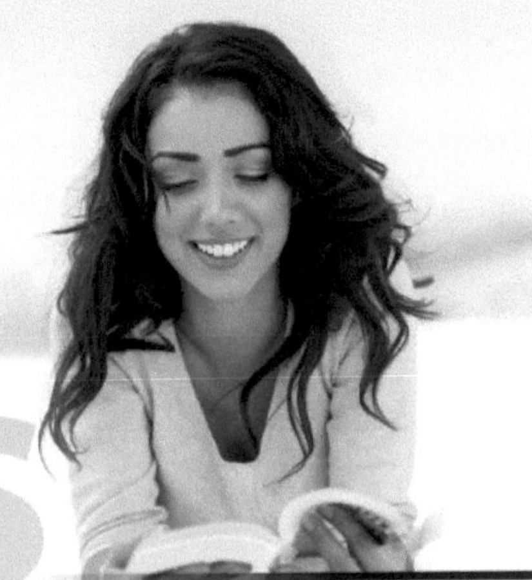

yes

I **want** morebooks!

Buy your books fast and straightforward online - at one of world's fastest growing online book stores! Environmentally sound due to Print-on-Demand technologies.

Buy your books online at
www.morebooks.shop

Kaufen Sie Ihre Bücher schnell und unkompliziert online – auf einer der am schnellsten wachsenden Buchhandelsplattformen weltweit! Dank Print-On-Demand umwelt- und ressourcenschonend produzi ert.

Bücher schneller online kaufen
www.morebooks.shop

info@omniscriptum.com
www.omniscriptum.com

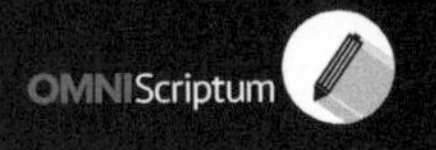

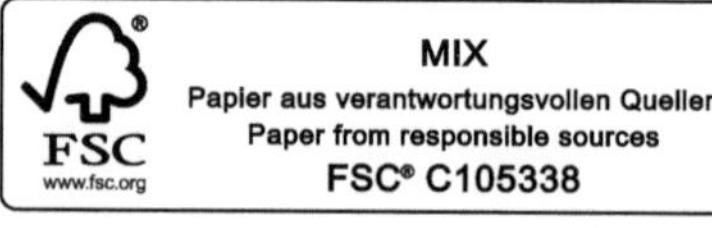

Printed by Books on Demand GmbH, Norderstedt / Germany